Breast Cancer's Silver Lining

What You Need to Know
About Your Reconstructive Options

WWW.MYRECONOPTIONS.COM

By Bernadette Hanson, RN

McClure ™
publishing

Bloomingdale, IL

ISBN-13: 978-0-9833697-2-1

ISBN-10: 0-9833697-2-0

LCCN: 2011939430

Cover Design and Interior Layout by Kathy McClure
www.mcclurepublishing.com

To order additional copies, please contact:
McClure Publishing, Inc.
800.659.4908
mcclurepublishing@msn.com

A percentage of the proceeds of this book will be donated to the Y-Me.org. They are a Chicago-based national nonprofit organization founded in 1978 with the mission to ensure, through information, empowerment and peer support, that no one faces breast cancer alone.

About Y-ME

Y-ME is the only place in the world a breast cancer patient – from the day of diagnosis throughout the course of their disease – can call 24/7 and speak to a peer, a breast cancer survivor who understands the physical and emotional challenges breast cancer patients face. For over 30 years, Y-ME has had a single mission – to assure, through information, empowerment, and peer support, that no one faces breast cancer alone. Our peer counselors are available 24 hours a day, 7 days a week, 365 days a year, in over 150 languages, through our toll-free Hotline.

Talk to a peer counselor at 1-800-221-2141, or visit y-me.org.

"Bernadette has bottled the essence of knowledge, insight and caring in this incredibly informative and fact filled book that will help all patients along their journey through a very difficult point in their lives."

David H. Song, MD, MBA, FACS
Professor and Vice-Chairman of Surgery
Chief of Plastic and Reconstructive Surgery

Disclaimer

The entire content of this book is not in any way meant to be medical advice or to replace any medical advice given by any member of your medical team. This book is simply information that may be used to start conversations with your plastic surgeon to help you to choose breast reconstructive options that are right for you.

CONTENTS

Introduction

Written from a nursing perspective, this is a user friendly, informational reference book for all those who have been diagnosed with breast cancer, those who are caretakers for someone who has been diagnosed with breast cancer and/or know someone with breast cancer.

There is a lot of information out there about breast cancer and breast reconstructive surgery, but not all of it is accurate and the last thing you need right now is erroneous information, confusion and frustration as you sift through this trying to sort out the facts from fiction regarding reconstruction.

This book will outline and take you through the most common breast reconstruction options. It will answer many of your questions as to whether a particular option is a good choice for you, what insurance covers, the benefits, restrictions and type of recovery you can expect for the different options available. It will talk about the difference between immediate and delayed reconstruction and the difference between reconstructions for a mastectomy as opposed to a lumpectomy.

It will further direct you to well established and trustworthy websites and support groups that can answer questions not addressed here. It will guide you as to the most important questions you need to ask your Plastic Surgeon and what specific information you need to have before deciding on your particular reconstruction.

My hope is that you will gain a better understanding and valuable insights that will equip and empower you on your breast reconstruction journey.

This book is dedicated to the millions of brave sisters in this world who have not let their breast cancer diagnosis define them and rule their lives, but who have gone on to live out their "New Normal", pink warriors taking a stand and waging their own war to overcome a common enemy.

You have my love, my support, my prayers and my respect.

Dear Reader,

You do not have this book in your hands by accident. Maybe you have just been diagnosed with breast cancer, or you are a caretaker for someone who has been diagnosed, or you know someone who has been diagnosed. You are about to gain knowledge that will become the "silver lining" in your situation.

Please take your time when reading this book. Personally, I can't read without a pen to underline and take notes and I have a tendency to dog ear my favorite pages.

There's a lot of information here that is very useful when speaking with your surgeons. Doctor appointments often are too brief, so bring your WRITTEN questions and don't hesitate to ask for clarification.

You are taking a giant step forward in the battle by being proactive and arming yourself with the basic information needed to jump start your conversations with your surgeons.

You are already headed in the direction of your "New Normal" where there are possibilities, choices and hope.

A Word about the Cover of This Book

I would like you to take note of the cover of this book. The visual images have a special significance for the breast cancer survivor.

You will notice that the scene depicted is one of the Sun breaking through storm clouds. When you are diagnosed with cancer, it can seem as though a dark cloud has settled over your life. It threatens with oppressive darkness and thunderous noises. You may feel like you're in a bleak and unfamiliar place, a place where you have no control and no idea of how long this ominous condition may last. You are thrust into a medical world for treatment where the language is foreign and the procedures can be distressing.

The truth is that every cloud has a "silver lining" and the storm will not last forever. It came to pass and did not come to stay. It is true that the darkest time is right before the dawn. In actuality, clouds do move quite fast and the sun is right there waiting to break through. The "silver lining" that represents breast reconstructive surgery is all about the choices and possibilities that await as you discover that there is life after breast cancer, that you can choose to have a "new normal", that you may even look and feel better after having your reconstruction than you did when you were first diagnosed with breast cancer.

I challenge you to face your storm with hope and courage as you discover your own personal breast reconstruction "silver lining".

Section 1

Proactive Steps to Take
Regarding Your Breasts

There are some steps that you can take on your own to be proactive regarding the health of your breasts. I cannot stress enough how important it is to do a monthly self-breast exam. No one knows the contours and regular features of your breast like you do. This is easily done after showering; feel both breasts to make sure there are no lumps or hard areas.

You are also looking at the skin of the breast to make sure there are no red areas, no blood tinged or foul smelling nipple discharge, no swelling, no dimpling, no painful areas.

If you find something, make an appointment with either your primary care physician or gynecologist. Get checked as soon as possible.

Make it a regular habit to have your annual mammogram after age 30; schedule it to coincide with some other annual occasion such as your birthday so you will not forget. It is **not** okay to skip a year, especially if there is a family history of breast or other cancers.

The good news is that more women are finding their own breast cancer earlier because they are being proactive and early detection is the key to early treatment, which means living out your long and healthy life.

A Word about Plastic and
Reconstructive Surgery

Be honest, when you hear the words, "plastic surgery", do you think about Hollywood stars, breast augmentations (making the breasts bigger using implants), nose jobs, face lifts, tummy tucks ... vain people with money trying to retain a youthful look ? I am not in any way demeaning cosmetic surgery, but simply asking you to look at and rethink your current understanding because while it is true that plastic surgeons are trained in cosmetic procedures, there's a whole other side that you need to know about. That is the reconstructive side of plastic surgery.

The word plastic actually comes from the Greek "plastikos", which means to reform, remold, restore, redefine, reconstruct, reshape, remodel. Plastic surgeons reconstruct malformed, injured, lost and missing parts of the body due to birth defects, congenital deformities, disease process (cancer, necrotizing fasciitis, etc.), burns and trauma (accidents). Their patients can range in age from newborns to senior citizens. Are you seeing the bigger picture now? This **is** why you see a plastic surgeon when you are diagnosed with breast cancer.

Repeat after me, "Reconstructing my breasts has NOTHING to do with vanity, but is simply replacing what cancer has taken away." I want you to repeat this as many times as you need to until you firmly believe it.

Women, as a whole, are nurturers and caretakers. We tend to put everything and everyone on the front burner and leave ourselves on the back burner. We will pour out, sacrifice, compromise, put our needs on hold and otherwise look to and take care of ourselves last. If you have been diagnosed with breast cancer, it's time to reset (temporarily) your priorities.

First and foremost, you need a plan and a medical team to address your cancer. Most major hospitals now have a holistic approach to your care. This means that they will probably have in place a team that will evaluate and plan the specific treatment needed for your individual case. On this team you will typically find: breast surgeons (they perform mastectomies and lumpectomies), radiologists (they take and interpret images/x-rays), pathologists (they look at tissue and fluid samples), oncologists (they will plan any necessary chemotherapy treatments), radiation oncologists (they will plan any radiation needed), genetic counselors (they determine whether you would benefit from genetic, BRCA, testing and among other things consider your personal genetic history and risks), social workers (they will evaluate your home support system and logistics needed), and last, but not least, plastic surgeons (they will reconstruct the breasts).

There is also a new trend that includes having a psycho-oncologist. This person's valuable contribution is to help someone, psychologically, through the breast cancer process. Someone who has been diagnosed with breast cancer may feel any or all of the following: anger (why me), guilt (I knew better than to smoke), fear (will I live to see my children grow up), depression (why bother with treatment, so many in my family have died of cancer), mourning (I am going to lose a very important part of who I am). There is absolutely no shame in asking for this type of help.

One of my favorite doctors put it like this ... if you had an infection you wouldn't hesitate to treat it. So, if you need someone to talk with and help you through the psychological issues, why would you hesitate to treat that? These are real conditions that can affect your physical health. People suffering from depression, fear, anxiety, etc. tend to have longer recovery times and more complications, as a whole. This can be treated just as sure as the cancer, so please do make good use of this resource.

A Few Basics before We Begin

I would like to make sure we are completely clear on a few things before we begin to discuss the actual reconstructive options.

Do you know the difference between a breast biopsy, a lumpectomy and a mastectomy in terms of what and how much tissue is removed from the breast?

A breast biopsy can be done either in the breast surgeon's office using ultra sound for exact specimen location and a needle and syringe for extracting a sample at the cancer site, or it may be done under a light sedative in an operating room using MRI imaging for guidance as to location with a surgical excision of the cancer site.

Another type of biopsy is called sentinel node. This may be done before or with a lumpectomy or mastectomy, in an operating room under anesthesia to see if the cancer has spread to the lymph nodes. Let me explain further,

> A lumpectomy is usually done in an operating room under general anesthesia and this involves taking a portion of the breast big enough to leave "clean" margins, (cancer cells are a measurable distance from the edge of the sample and not touching it so the margins are disease free). If the pathology results show that the margins are not "clean" a re-excision lumpectomy is often done.

Depending on how large the breast is and how large a specimen needs to be taken, this can leave a deficit or indentation.

A partial mastectomy is removing a portion of breast tissue that is equal to approximately one fourth or 25% of your breast. It is a larger portion than a lumpectomy, which removes lumps and surrounding tissue and a smaller portion than a mastectomy which removes all breast tissue.

A mastectomy can be simple, meaning the all (inner) breast tissue is removed as well as the areola and nipple, or radical or modified radical, meaning that all the (inner) breast tissue, again including the areola and nipple, is removed as well as lymph nodes and other surrounding tissues. It can be skin sparing, meaning that the breast surgeon leaves as much (outer) breast skin as possible to give the plastic surgeon more to work with. Mastectomies also may be nipple sparing, please talk to your breast surgeon for a recommendation for your individual situation.

Another type of mastectomy is called completion. Your breast surgeon would remove all remaining (inner) breast tissue as well as the areola and nipple, if needed. This happens when a lumpectomy has been done previously and now full reconstruction of the breast is desired, so all breast tissue needs to be removed. This may also be done in cases of recurrent cancer or when more lumpectomy excisions are needed to get a clean margin.

The amount of actual breast tissue removed greatly impacts the type of reconstruction that will be done. You can imagine that reconstructing the smaller deficit from a lumpectomy would be different from reconstructing the larger area created from having a mastectomy.

Your breast surgeon will send these samples to pathology in order to determine your "staging". This means the tissue will be examined to find out exactly what type of cancer it is and how far it has spread.

Staging is essential to the reconstructive process as it determines the treatment that will be given for the cancer. Depending on what treatment is necessary, (chemotherapy, radiation, and more procedures by your breast surgeon); your reconstruction may be delayed. I'd like to stress here that your whole team is unified and works together to first and foremost treat the cancer and this certainly includes your plastic surgeon.

IMMEDIATE VS. DELAYED RECONSTRUCTION

Let's talk about the difference between immediate and delayed reconstruction. Immediate reconstruction is when the first stage of reconstruction is performed at the same surgery as your mastectomy and delayed reconstruction, is when this is done as a separate surgery after your mastectomy and/or treatment and the reasons why each would happen. We'll also look at oncoplastic reconstruction.

Immediate reconstruction has some distinct advantages. Your plastic surgeon can make good use of the pliant, elastic breast skin after the mastectomy. This is helpful no matter which type of reconstruction is being done. You will wake up after surgery with a new breast mound as opposed to a flat chest which may be a psychological as well as physiological benefit for you. You will have an acceptable appearance in clothing right away. You will already be moving forward towards your "new normal" upon discharge from the hospital.

Delayed reconstruction may happen because you are so overwhelmed at the time of your breast cancer diagnosis that you just want to address the disease first and have time to process before going on to have reconstruction. This is perfectly fine. The cancer absolutely **MUST** be addressed; the reconstruction is a choice and can be done at a later date. In the meantime, you can choose to have a breast prosthesis custom made just for you to fit in a special bra that will give you symmetry while wearing clothing. Yes, this prosthesis is covered by insurance and I'll bet you're asking if your insurance would cover delayed reconstruction as well. The answer to that is, YES, as the law is written at the time of this writing. More about insurance coverage later.

Another reason the reconstruction may be delayed is that, because of your particular staging, you need more treatment to take care of the cancer. You may need chemotherapy, which can last from weeks to months. Chemo fights your disease, but it also weakens your immune system. Your body needs to heal and recover from chemo before you assault it with more surgery. Exams and blood tests will be done by your oncologist to make sure your body is strong enough to withstand reconstructive surgery. There is usually a four week, or so, delay period from the end of your chemo until the time you will be able to have reconstruction. The exact delay time will be determined by your oncologist.

You may have needed radiation therapy. This can also last from weeks to a month, or so, as determined by your radiation oncologist. Radiation creates some specific and difficult problems for the reconstructive surgeon. It can create some pretty harsh changes in your skin, scar tissue, skin thickening, color changes, skin sensitivities, loss of elasticity, all of which could be challenges when reconstructing the breast, but there are some great options and solutions, as well. On average, the delay time between your last radiation treatment and your reconstructive surgery is six months. This gives your skin time to heal and soften to optimize your final reconstructive results. You may be wondering if having radiation will limit your reconstructive options. This is really determined on an individual basis as not everyone reacts to radiation the same way. I will tell you this, I have seen every type of reconstruction done on radiated breasts, and the best results are the work of the more skilled, experienced and highly trained plastic surgeons. It can and has been done.

Oncoplastic reconstruction happens when the plastic surgeon is involved in breast conservation therapy such as a lumpectomy or partial mastectomy. During this surgery either the breast tissue is rearranged or local tissues are recruited (back skin and fat, etc.) to fill in/replace what has been removed. Not only does this give you optimal results regarding the shape and appearance of the breast that is conserved, but also offers symmetry needed to balance the other breast.

This is a relatively new kind of reconstruction. It's especially helpful when it's been determined that radiation treatment will be necessary. The cleft or space left from the removal of tissue will, at first, be filled with fluid. This inflammatory response is your body's normal reaction to surgery and will actually look like little or no tissue has been removed, but as this resolves and the fluid is absorbed by your body, the deficit may be noticeable depending on the location and amount of tissue actually taken out. Add radiation to the mix and now you have skin that will shrink into this space and become tough, inflexible and difficult to correct. Not impossible, but difficult. Think of putting shrink wrap over a fish bowl and sucking out the air, which is similar to how food is vacuum packed and sealed. Unless that tissue is rearranged, you can see there will be an obvious deformity.

A Word about Prophylactic Mastectomies

A prophylactic mastectomy is a preemptive, proactive decision to have the noncancerous breast removed in an effort to prevent disease from occurring there in the future.

Are you asking yourself why anyone would ask to have a perfectly healthy breast surgically removed? There are many good reasons to do just that.

Here are a few:

Someone may have a very strong family history of cancer in general. These may be varied types of cancers that have occurred on either the Dad's (Paternal) or Mom's (Maternal) side of the family. Or, maybe there is a history of breast cancer in several immediate family members, your Grandmother, your Mother, or your sister. Or, you may be so anxious and worried about the possibility of the cancer recurring in the non-cancer breast that it literally preoccupies your thoughts and affects your quality of life. Often times, the breast team member from genetics or cancer risk will advise this person to take a BRCA test to see if they test positive for the breast cancer gene.

Knowing whether you are positive for, or carry this gene, may be the deciding factor when choosing to have the noncancerous breast removed because now you know that you may be pre-disposed to getting cancer again, this time in the other breast. Your cancer risk team member can explain to you, percentage wise, exactly what your individual results mean for you. Knowing that you carry the gene is also significant as far as the possibility that your daughters or sons and granddaughters or grandsons may carry the gene, as well. There are many women who have not been diagnosed with breast cancer, but simply test positive for the BRCA gene and elect to have prophylactic bilateral (both sides) mastectomies.

There are also some good reasons to **not** have a prophylactic mastectomy. The number one reason to keep your noncancerous breast is because, let's face it, it's healthy … why disturb healthy tissue? There's no risk like no risk and when it comes to surgery, the more surgical sites you have, the more recovery you will have to endure. The more scarring there will be, the more potential for infection, bleeding, etc. (all the common risks of any surgical procedure).

Another major reason to keep your healthy breast is to preserve erogenous sensation. This is probably the last thing on your mind right now, especially if you are newly diagnosed, but believe me when I tell you this, a mastectomy will remove all breast tissue, including the areola and nipple and all the sensations connected to them. Your plastic surgeon will be well able to reconstruct a great looking nipple, but it will not have erogenous sensation. You may be able to differentiate between hot, cold and pressure, but you will lose the ability to be aroused that you have with a normal nipple. This cannot be undone, so please consider carefully.

All of this has been said to come to this conclusion, if you have been diagnosed with breast cancer in one breast, you will, at some point, be asked to think about the possibility of removing the other (noncancerous) breast and this does play into your reconstructive options.

The way this decision affects reconstruction is mainly related to the specific type of reconstruction you desire and how that works with the tissue you have available for your plastic surgeon to work with. Obviously, it will take more to reconstruct two breasts as opposed to one and a lady who has a more slender body type will have less excess tissue to offer than one who has a more generous body type.

Let's Talk About Insurance Coverage

Are you ready for some really good news? In 1998, a federal law was signed into effect called the **Women's Health & Cancer Rights Act.** In effect, it states that an insurance provider that offers coverage and benefits for a mastectomy **shall provide** coverage and benefits for not only reconstructing **the breast on which the mastectomy was performed, but also the other breast** for symmetry procedures. Symmetry procedures are surgeries that address the non-cancerous breast to make it more symmetrical or similar in size/volume, shape and projection to the breast that had the mastectomy and reconstruction. This usually happens at the second stage of reconstruction and is done by making it either bigger (augmentation usually with an implant), smaller (doing a reduction) or lifting (doing a mastopexy). Other services mandated to be covered are; prosthesis and complications of a mastectomy including lymphedemas. See below:

Signed into Law on October 21, 1998 - ASPS is working with federal regulators as they draft guidance on implementation of the new law.

Sec. 901. Short Title.

This title may be cited as the "Women's Health and Cancer Rights Act of 1998".

Sec. 902. Amendments to the Employee Retirement Income Security Act of 1974.

(a) **In General** - Subpart B of part 7 of subtitle B of title I of the Employee Retirement Income Security Act of 1974 (29 U.S.C. 1185 *et seq.*) is amended by adding at the end the following new section:

Sec. 713. Required Coverage for Reconstructive Surgery Following Mastectomies.

(a) **In General** - A group health plan, and a health insurance issuer providing health insurance coverage in connection with a group health plan, that provides medical and surgical benefits with respect to a mastectomy shall provide, in a case of a participant or beneficiary who is receiving benefits in connection with a mastectomy and who elects breast reconstruction in connection with such mastectomy, coverage for:

- Reconstruction of the breast on which the mastectomy has been performed;
- Surgery and reconstruction of the other breast to produce a symmetrical appearance;
- Prostheses and physical complications all stages of mastectomy, including lymphedemas; in a manner determined in consultation with the attending physician and the patient. Such coverage may be subject to annual deductibles and coinsurance provisions as may be deemed appropriate and as are consistent with those established for other benefits under the plan or coverage. Written notice of the availability of such coverage shall be delivered to the participant upon enrollment and annually thereafter.

Is this a silver lining, or what? Listed below are some websites to verify this law, but I'd also like you to search or Google, "1998 Federal Breast Reconstruction Law".

Now, your insurance carrier will cover both breast reconstruction for the breast with cancer and the opposite breast symmetry procedures according to your particular plan. If you have a 70/30 plan or an 80/20 plan, etc., that is how it will be covered. I'd like to mention here that not all facilities accept all insurances, so once you've found your breast team and plastic surgeon, make sure that the hospital that the doctors are associated with accepts your plan and the doctors are in your network. A call to either your insurance company or the Insurance Department of the hospital you're interested in can better answer your questions.

As promised, here are the websites to verify this wonderful law:

www.dol.gov/ebsa/publications/whcra.html

www.breastcenter.com/support/rights.php

www.plasticsurgery.org/reconstructive-procedures

Please note, to explore the plastic surgery site, you need to type in "1998 federal breast reconstruction law" in the search box.

A Few More Things To Consider

Whether you decide on breast reconstruction using autologous tissue (tissue from other sites on your own body) or implant reconstruction (usually a two stage process using tissue expanders first), on average, the entire process from the initial surgery to tattooing and nipple reconstruction takes about twelve months. After your last procedure you will generally see your plastic surgeon yearly for an evaluation of your reconstruction.

The common sequence will go something like this the initial surgery will create a breast "mound". This will need to heal and have the swelling that is created by surgery resolve. This part can take eight to twelve weeks. The second stage will address symmetry procedures (the augmentation, reduction or mastopexy discussed earlier) for the non-cancer breast as well as revision or adjustment/alteration of the reconstructed breast mound. Again, there will be an eight to twelve week period of post-op healing. Once the two breasts are symmetrical, notice I did not say "perfect" as **all** women have some degree of asymmetry, one of my favorite doctors says that they are sisters, not twins.

Now you are ready for the last two procedures which include tattooing, then an eight week healing time and, finally, nipple reconstruction. Some doctors prefer to do the nipple reconstruction first and then the tattooing, this is a matter of preference as I have seen both methods produce very good results.

The medical micro-pigmentation or areola and nipple tattooing will be an outpatient procedure often done in the clinic, usually just with a local anesthetic to the site. Yes, you guessed it, the machine used to tattoo it is very similar to one used in regular tattoo parlors. Some major differences are; in the clinic there is more privacy, the technique and sterilization process are regulated by the facility, insurance will cover this as a medical procedure related to breast cancer.

Nipple reconstruction is also an outpatient procedure and again, usually done in the clinic with local anesthetic to the site. Some doctors take skin to create the nipple from other sites (inner thigh, the other nipple, etc). I've seen my doctors use the skin that is right where the normal nipple has been removed, make some incisions, some suturing, some remodeling and create the nipple. Think of it as "skin origami". This does create quite an acceptable result. Often, the nipple will be made larger than the intended result because it will shrink somewhat (atrophy).

You may opt to not have the last two procedures, and that's okay. If you change your mind, it can be done at a later date. I'd like you to consider the following, picture a face without a nose. It's still a face, but when you add the nose; it becomes much more esthetically appealing and recognizable as a face, doesn't it? It works the same way when you add the nipple and tattooing to your reconstructed breast. It becomes much more realistic and normal looking.

I'd also like you to be aware that an "illusion" nipple can be done instead of a reconstructed nipple. This is when the nipple is tattooed on in a 3D illusion pattern that gives the "optical illusion" of a raised nipple out of clothing. I'll bet you're wondering why someone would opt for that. The reconstructed nipple will have all the features of a normal nipple **except** that it will always be erect as the muscles that allow the nipple to contract and relax have been removed when the mastectomy is done. An easy solution for this is to cover them when wearing close fitting garments or swimsuits with a nursing pad, which can be found in any drug store. I have also seen some other creative solutions, including a product called "nippits" that can be found online.

What About Scarring?

Surgery is, in essence, planned injury. Any time your body is injured, it has a defense mechanism called the inflammatory response that springs into action. Fluids, nutrients and antibodies from your body's natural defense system, called the immune system, will all converge upon the injured area to heal and repair any damage. The physical results that are manifested are; swelling, itching, pain, redness and scabbing (your body's way of sealing off leaks and protecting the site from infection). The marks left as a result of this healing process are scars. Scar tissue can be above or below the skin. It can be tough, red, raised, tender to touch and quite unsightly.

Plastic surgeons, as a whole, are very careful as to placement, length and pattern of the surgical incisions they make. They will usually try to hide the scar lines in other natural lines already present, if this is possible. They use special sutures and closing techniques in an effort to keep scarring to a minimum, but the fact is, if you have surgery, it is inevitable that you will have some degree of scarring.

There are many commercial products available that claim to "erase" scars. I have also seen claims that there are magical laser treatments for scars. I have not seen anyone achieve the exact "miracle" results that are promised by these products and treatments. What I have seen and what has been documented by several scar studies, is that scars will usually take a regimented course over a year's time where the worst stage will be seen around the seventh month and will get incrementally better from there to about the twelfth month when you will see the scar soften, flatten and get lighter in color. How much better will it actually get? The best indicator would be to look at the scars you have now. Just remember that even if you have the world's best plastic surgeon, some other limiting factors are how you are wired genetically in regards to scarring and how well the surgical site is taken care of in the post-op period.

What are some of the risks related to surgery?

We've covered some of the benefits related to having breast reconstruction surgery. What about the risks? In general, there are risks of simply having anesthesia (nausea, sore throat, reaction to medications used, etc.), infection, bleeding, pain, need for further procedures, hematoma (blood collection under the skin at the surgery site), seroma (fluid collection under the skin at the surgery site), scarring, injury to other structures including; tissues, blood vessels or nerves and wound healing complications.

In addition, and specific to having reconstructive surgery using autologous flaps (your own tissues), risks also include; inability to perform flap due to unusual anatomical anomalies (blood vessels needed are not available/accessible or suitable to support flap), partial or complete loss of flap due to clotting off of blood vessels used to connect flap to the chest. These surgeries are done under a microscope using suture that is smaller in diameter than a single strand of hair. There may be abdominal bulges or hernias, breast asymmetry, and wound healing complications at the surgical site.

Risks specific to having breast reconstruction surgery using tissue expanders and implants are, in addition to the general risks above, loss of either tissue expander or implant due to infection, capsular contracture (this is hardening of the area inside the breast around the implant or tissue expander), or exposure (this is where an area of skin opens and the tissue expander or implant can be seen).

Other risks include; obesity (having an excess of more than 30% body fat), diabetes (in general affects wound healing), hypertension (important to be under control in order to prevent clots during surgery), history of radiation to area (as discussed earlier), smoking (nicotine is a blood vessel constrictor and restricts healing blood flow), heart conditions (it must be healthy enough to withstand the stresses/amount of time involved in surgery).

Wow ... that's a lot to take in. Is it still worth it to undergo breast reconstruction surgery considering all the possible risks, ABSOLUTELY.

What if your doctor had to get your consent to walk across the street? He would have to explain all the possible risks, correct? You may fall off the curb, you may get hit by an oncoming car, you may slip on the sidewalk, there may be nearby construction with a risk of having an accident associated with what was going on there, the traffic light may not be working, and on and on, but I'll bet you'll walk across the street carefully, inherently knowing these risks anyway. Your doctor will discuss the risks and complications of your surgery, not to alarm or frighten you , but to educate and prepare you for these possibilities.

NOTES

Section 2

Two Basic Kinds of Breast Reconstruction

The two basic types of breast reconstruction are 1) autologous flap or using your own tissue as a donor site and 2) implants. There is also breast reconstruction using a combination of flaps and implants. More about this type later. Let's look at the pros and cons of the two basic types of reconstruction.

Flap reconstruction uses your own skin and fat and can be taken from a variety of places or donor sites. Depending on your individual anatomy, medical history, priorities, and preferences and, of course, a physical exam by your plastic surgeon, possible donor sites are; the lower abdomen (hip to hip from just under your belly button/umbilicus to above the pubis area), the upper back area, the inner thighs, or the buttocks. To simplify, let's discuss one of the most requested types of flap reconstruction, the abdominal or DIEP flap (deep inferior epigastric perforator).

The pros of using your own abdominal tissue are; "silver lining." You can have your own skin and fat relocated from where you don't want it (abdomen), to where you do want it (breast). Who wouldn't absolutely love going up a cup size and down a pants size with the added bonus of a flat tummy? Now, we're talking real benefits! Now, if in the future, you gain or lose weight your reconstructed breast tissue (which has no idea it is no longer on your abdomen because of an internal mechanism called memory retention) will gain or lose weight as if it were still on your abdomen ... gain weight, breast gets bigger ...

lose weight, breast gets smaller. This is why if you do not have enough tissue for this surgery, it makes no sense to globally gain weight because after you have this lovely breast surgically created and now want to lose the weight you gained that was not on your stomach, your new breast will also lose volume as you lose weight.

How big, exactly, will this breast created by using the abdominal skin and fat be? Let's do a little test. Look at the skin and fat on your abdomen from hip to hip and from your umbilicus (belly button) to just above the pubis bone. Pinch it. This is what your plastic surgeon has to work with. (The upper abdomen is not used in this type of reconstruction.) How does it compare to the size of your breast? If you are thinking about bilateral reconstruction, divide this in half to get an idea of how much is available for each side.

Continuing on with the pros; this is a better match for the opposite breast that has a natural droop or ptosis. This tissue is very pliable and can be made to look very natural or can be lifted according to what you'd like done on the other breast. If you've been wanting to get both breasts lifted or reduced, here's your golden opportunity. If you are happy with the look of your natural aging breasts, this can easily be accomplished. This is the choice you should discuss with your plastic surgeon. This is your own natural tissue; rejection by your body is slim to none. Once this heals, it's yours for life, no replacements needed (in contrast to implants). The procedure done on your abdomen is very similar to the cosmetic procedure done during a $20,000.00 abdoplasty/tummy tuck.

Same scar pattern, same closure, same end result ... "silver lining"! The difference between the cosmetic procedure and the medical procedure is that in the cosmetic procedure the skin and fat is disposed of or thrown away.

There are some cons to using your abdomen; surgery is approximately six hours for one breast and twelve hours for two breasts. There is a hospital stay afterwards of three to five days and a post-op recovery period of four to six weeks. There are incisions on the breast area and the abdomen; so consequently, there will be healing, scars and risks of potential complications on both the breast and abdomen. This donor site can only be utilized once, so you need to have made a firm decision as to whether you want to replace one breast (unilateral) or two (bilateral). You can still choose to have a prophylactic mastectomy and reconstruction at a different time, but since the abdomen donor site has already been used, the other breast will need to use a different donor site. I have seen very nice results when this has been done, especially when it's been done by a plastic surgeon with experience in this particular area of matching breasts and creating symmetry with two different donor site areas.

Tissue expander/implant reconstruction uses either a silicone gel or saline filled implant to reconstruct your breast. Usually the first stage will be placement of a tissue expander (an empty breast shaped shell with a silver dollar sized metallic port), often with an acellular dermal matrix to support the lower pole of the reconstruction. This dermal matrix is processed and purified donated skin that is free from cells that can cause inflammation or rejection and that literally assimilates into normal tissue. The upper part of the tissue expander is placed under your chest muscle, think of the acellular dermal matrix as a kind of sling or hammock holding and supporting the bottom half of the tissue expander.

Saline is added to this expander in the weeks following your mastectomy, often done as a quick nurse visit in the clinic, increasing volume and allowing the breast skin to stretch as your new breast is shaped, formed and increased week by week. When the desired volume is achieved, there will be an exchange surgery to remove the tissue expander and replace it with a permanent silicone gel or saline implant.

A quick word about silicone gel versus saline for the permanent implant. After a mastectomy, there is no breast tissue present; imagine an empty shell that needs to be filled. When discussing the two types of implants, it would be very helpful to actually hold them in your hand as you are talking to your plastic surgeon. Every plastics office I've been to has these sample implants just for this purpose. Pinch the top of each type and let it hang. You will notice that the saline implant will display a rippling or wrinkled appearance. It's just the nature of the chemistry of saline solution and how it displaces in this particular container (the implant shell). This is what will be seen under your breast skin. It works very well when used in a cosmetic augmentation because there is breast skin **and** tissue in front of it. After a mastectomy there is no breast tissue to cover the rippling and it will be apparent.

Now, as you hold the saline implant, move it back and forth a little. You will be moving your chest, right? Did you hear or feel some sloshing around? Just want to make sure you realize some things up front. I want you to do the same tests to the gel implant. Do you notice how similar the consistency is to natural breast tissue? Don't hesitate to put an article of clothing over the gel implant and feel how realistic it is. This is how it will look and feel under your breast skin.

I can hear some of you reading this thinking and disputing if gel implants are safe — what if it ruptures, right? It is true that if a saline implant ruptures, the saline will most likely be absorbed by your body. Most of you probably remember the big scare regarding gel implants in the 1980's. That was actually a good thing because it caused the companies that make implants to develop a good product into a better product. Truth be told, there was not one solid documented case of any gel implant directly causing any untoward effect or disease. There simply is no convincing scientific support to the claims made against the safety of the gel implant.

Here are some things you need to know about gel implants, one of the improvements was to replace the liquid gel content with a thick cohesive (gummy bear-like) content. If the argument is indeed, about the safety of silicone, why are the outer shells of both the saline and gel implants made of the same silicone? The fact is, when the gel implants were taken off the market for a short time and not used for cosmetic augmentations, they were still allowed to be used for breast cancer patients. Does it make sense to allow this particular group of women to use an "unsafe" product and intentionally put them in harm's way?

Physiologically, your body protects itself against foreign objects by creating a shell or capsule around anything implanted. For instance, a pacemaker, a joint replacement and certainly breast implants. So, even if there is a break or rupture in the implant, it will usually stay within this capsule. I've witnessed a couple of interesting demonstrations regarding the difficulty of rupturing the gel implant. I've seen a gel implant run over by a truck and retain its integrity, and I've also seen a gel implant hurled at lightning speed into a wall and not suffer any damage. I am simply encouraging you to do some research on your own before dismissing the possibility of having gel implants placed.

Here are some pros of using implant reconstruction; the surgery is approximately one hour per breast, this is an outpatient procedure if done by itself and an overnight stay if done with a mastectomy, post-op recovery is two weeks, the incisions and subsequent healing and scarring is only on the breasts. Within reason, you can pick your size. If you were a "B" cup and have always desired to be a "C" cup or even a small "D" cup, now is your chance. Your new size is dependent on how well your skin will stretch out. At the exchange surgery (removal of the tissue expander and placement of the permanent gel implant), your plastic surgeon can use an implant for your other breast to augment (make it bigger) for symmetry ... "silver lining". This type of breast reconstruction is also a very good choice if you have a slender body type and no really good donor sites to offer, or if you do have several donor sites and simply cannot make up your mind and you want to move forward. This is a great choice because you still preserve all your other options, or if you don't have the time to invest for a lengthy post-op recovery right now, go for the implants and later, yes, even years later, come back and have the implants removed and an autologous flap reconstruction done.

I can almost hear you asking if insurance will pay for that because you've already had some reconstruction done. The answer to that is, "YES MA'AM." Another interesting fact is that if you lose or gain weight, your reconstruction stays exactly the same size and does not fluctuate when your weight does.

Some cons to implant reconstruction are; you will need weekly visits to the clinic for expansion, your plastic surgeon is placing a foreign body in you and this means you have to be careful for signs of capsular contracture (where the capsule around the implant contracts and causes tightness, pain and wrinkling), infection and exposure. You may need revisions and you will need replacements as the average life of an implant is ten to fifteen years. Unless you have a bilateral mastectomy with bilateral implant reconstruction (which is a very close match), it's more challenging to match the opposite breast because of the natural tendency towards ptosis (drooping). Even if the non-cancer breast has an implant, there is some breast tissue present and it will succumb to gravity.

Let's talk about the combination surgeries that use both your own tissue and an implant. This would usually involve the skin and fat from your upper back area, the LAT (using skin, fat and some muscle) or the TAP (same area as the LAT except no muscle is used). A tissue expander is placed under this tissue and you will go on to have weekly fills and subsequent exchange surgery to place the gel implant. This surgery gives a very natural looking mound and still allows you to determine the size you'd like to be (within reason) because of the flexibility of having the expander.

So, looking at the advantages and disadvantages of both using your own tissues (autologous reconstruction) and using the two stage implant reconstruction, there is a lot to think about. One of my favorite doctors explains it this way, consider renting versus owning. Autologous reconstruction is like owning ... you make a big investment up front, but then you own it, it's yours for life. The big investment involves more surgery, more healing, more scar sites, more recovery time and then your breast is yours for life.

The two stage implant reconstruction is more like renting. There is less invested up front and you do not own / keep it forever. As mentioned earlier, the average life span of an implant is ten to fifteen years. So, you will, over the span of your life have several implants replaced. The time spent in surgery is much less, scar sites are only on the breasts and healing and recovery time is less.

SOME INFORMATION YOU NEED BEFORE DECIDING ON AN OPTION

Think about your priorities as far as:

- Do you just want to treat the cancer right now and make a decision regarding reconstruction later ... maybe how your body looks in and out of clothing is not a priority right now, or is it a priority to look good in clothing, or is your priority to look good out of clothing?

- Consider whether you desire immediate or delayed reconstruction.

- Reflect on whether you would like to use your own tissues, implants, or a combination of both.

- Give some time to really think about having some type of surgery on the non-cancer breast, whether that would be either a symmetry procedure or a prophylactic mastectomy.

Remember, if you have always desired to have a change in the shape, size or appearance of your breasts, this is the time, or would you prefer to stay the same size either with a natural droop (ptosis) or be lifted or would you like to be smaller or larger.

Think about your lifestyle and all the things happening in your life besides breast cancer. How much time can you commit to post-operative recovery?

NOTES

Section 3

Let's Look at Options

Let's look at the most popular, most requested, most common forms of breast reconstruction. This is by no means an exhaustive list and plastic surgeons have their own specialties and surgeries that they personally excel in. Variations of all of these types of reconstructions are also done, so please take time with your plastic surgeon and discuss the options best suited to your priorities, your body type and your preferences.

We'll look at autologous types of reconstruction, including combination of autologous and implant first and then the two stage implant reconstruction.

DIEP Flap Reconstruction

DIEP stands for deep inferior epigastric perforator, which simply describes the name of the main blood vessel that provides profusion/blood flow for healing the tissue that will be used for the reconstruction. Skin, fat and blood vessels will be removed from the lower abdomen (hip to hip and from the belly button/umbilicus to the pubis bone) to recreate the breast. Typically no muscle or very little is removed.

Scars will be on the breast(s) in either a round or "football"/ elliptical shape and there will also be a line from hip to hip in a typical "tummy tuck"/ abdoplasty pattern.

This type of surgery is best suited for someone with enough lower abdominal tissue available and who is healthy enough to withstand the six hour (one side) to twelve hour (both sides) surgery time needed. This is not a good option for a person who smokes or has cardiac restrictions/conditions that would prohibit a lengthy surgery. This surgery is also not a good option for a very thin lady or someone who has excessive inner or outer abdominal scarring from past surgeries or inner tissue scarring from years of insulin use. Other contraindications are having a history of an emergency C-section delivery where abdominal structures that are needed for the DIEP may have been compromised or having had a cosmetic tummy tuck (abdoplasty) in the past.

There is an estimated three to five day hospital stay post-operatively. Recovery is approximately four weeks. There will be lifting restrictions on the arm of the side that is being reconstructed, typically no more than five pounds. This means that you will not be lifting dishes, vacuuming, pushing a grocery cart, doing the laundry, lifting arm weights, lifting small children, pushing a stroller or walking the dog.

You will have drains in both your abdomen (donor site) and in the reconstructed breast. Yes, you do need them, they are necessary to drain fluids, that occur as part of the inflammatory response we talked about earlier, from the body in order to prevent infection, as these fluids are a great medium for bacteria, and they also help keep swelling and, subsequently, pain to a minimum. Bet you're wondering how long you have to keep them in. Commonly they are not removed until the twenty-four hours total is 30cc's or less for two consecutive days. At this point your body will be able to absorb any more fluids that are formed. I'm going to give you a valuable tip here, the more you use your arms and the more active you are, in general, the more fluid you will produce and the longer the drains will stay in.

Post-op garments will be loose fitting tops or camisoles. You have just had micro surgery where your doctor has sewn together blood vessels with sutures that are about the diameter of a single piece of hair. The idea is to have the blood vessels heal together without pressure to avoid clotting or kinking which can lead to decreased or cessation of blood flow and subsequent loss of the breast flap. So, please keep the pressure off the surgical site. You will most likely be released to wear a bra in about four weeks post-operatively.

You will find in each reconstruction, that loose fitting garments are a requirement to help your body heal properly.

TUG Flap reconstruction

TUG stands for transverse upper gracilis and this describes the location of the flap which is your upper inner thigh. Skin and fat from your thigh is used to recreate your breast. Can you say ... "silver lining"?

Scars will be on the breast in either a round or elliptical/oval shape and in a straight line on the inner aspect of your thigh from mid-thigh to the area where your leg meets your lower body. Depending on the actual laxity or looseness of your thigh skin the scar may be either horizontal or vertical, VUG.

This type of surgery is best suited to someone who has enough thigh tissue to create the size of breast desired and who is healthy enough to withstand the six hour (one side) to twelve hour (both sides) surgery. This is not a good option for someone who may have scarring in this area, such as is seen in hidradenitis, which is a condition of overactive sweat glands that rupture, drain and leave scars.

There is an estimated three to five day stay post operatively. The recovery time needed is about four weeks. There will be lifting restrictions on the arm of the side that is being reconstructed, typically no lifting of more than five pounds. There are also restrictions with regard to sitting; using the restroom is fine, otherwise the leg should be straight and kept elevated as much as possible to minimize swelling.

An extra bonus with this surgery is, if you have opted to have only one breast reconstructed, you may need to have liposuction done to the other thigh to create symmetry. This is typically done at the second stage surgery as deemed necessary by your plastic surgeon.

You will have drains in both the breast and the inner thigh (donor site); this can be a little cumbersome, but well worth it, considering the end results. Again, drains stay in until they are 30cc's or less per twenty-four hour period for at least two consecutive days.

Post-op garments will be loose tops or camisoles so the blood vessels and flap can heal without any pressure.

SGAP Flap Reconstruction

SGAP stands for superior gluteal artery perforator which describes the location of the blood vessels and tissue used for this surgery, that's right; it's the upper portion of your buttock.

Scars will be on the breast in either a round or elliptical/oval pattern and also in a straight horizontal line across the top of the buttock. The typical length of this scar is about four inches.

This surgery is best suited for someone who has enough tissue to recreate the breast and is healthy enough to withstand the six to eight hour surgery. If bilateral, meaning you desire that both of your breasts be reconstructed, this will usually be done in stages, one side first and then a healing period of about two months before the other side will be done. This is more challenging if done as a bilateral reconstruction and is more safely and easily done when staged. Try to imagine the intricacy of keeping everything together, harvesting a flap on one area and maintaining bleeding and closure and needing to transplant it to another part of the body that is located in an area where you have to turn the entire patient to access it.

This surgery is not a good option for someone who doesn't have enough tissue to offer or who prefers to not use the buttock area to recreate the breast.

There will be a three to five day stay afterwards with an approximate four week recovery period. Restrictions include no lifting of more than five pounds with the arm on the side of the reconstruction and minimal sitting. Using the restroom is fine, but you will need to be either lying down or standing for a couple of weeks as you heal.

Added bonus with this surgery is that if you opt to only have one breast reconstructed, you may need to have liposuction done to your other buttock for symmetry. This is usually done at the second stage surgery as deemed necessary by your plastic surgeon.

You will have drains both in the breast and in the buttock (donor site); again these are normally removed until the drainage total is 30cc's or less for twenty-four hours for two consecutive days.

Post-op garments will be loose tops or camisoles to allow the flaps to heal without pressure.

LAT and TAP Flap reconstruction

LAT stands for Latissimus flap which describes the back muscle where this flap is taken from. TAP, or Thoracodorsal artery perforator flap, is from the same area but differs from the LAT in that no muscle is taken and the skin and tissue is rotated around to the breast area to create the basic reconstructive mound. Both of these can include placement of a tissue expander, as well, and in that case, it would be considered a combination (autologous and implant) surgery.

Scars will be on the breast in either a round or elliptical/oval pattern and there will also be a line on the upper back area that can be placed at an angle either horizontally or vertically. Please let your plastic surgeon know your preference for scar placement. You may be someone who has occasion to wear a lot of evening gowns and would need placement to be hidden horizontally or maybe you wear clothing that would be better suited to having the scar line placed vertically. Yes, you can request this and your plastic surgeon will do their best to make this happen, depending on the exact location used.

This surgery is best suited to someone who wants a shorter surgery and recovery time and who does not mind scars on the upper back area. This is not the best choice for someone who is a professional golfer and rock climber as they may notice some decrease in muscle strength with the arm on the reconstructed side. This is seldom felt when the TAP reconstruction is done.

This surgery will usually have a twenty three hour to two day stay afterwards with a two to three week recovery period. If a tissue expander is placed you will be getting weekly fills at the clinic/office. This will entail coming to the clinic and having the nurse inject saline solution into the tissue expander on a weekly basis until you have reached your desired volume. Restrictions will be no lifting greater than five pounds on the side of the reconstruction.

You will have drains both in the breast and the back area (donor site). Again, they will stay until the drainage output is 30cc's or less per twenty-four hour period for two consecutive days.

Post-op garments will be loose tops or camisoles to allow for healing without pressure to the area.

Implant Reconstruction

This is generally a two stage process that involves placing a tissue expander first, followed by weekly fills with saline solution in the office/clinic, and then after the desired volume has been achieved, there is an exchange surgery where the tissue expander is removed and the gel implant is placed. The tissue expander is an empty breast shaped shell with a silver dollar sized metal port. Your doctor or nurse will use a magnetic port finder to locate the spot on the expander where saline solution can be injected. The breast skin over the port is generally numb after the mastectomy, and the weekly fill appointments usually take about ten to fifteen minutes.

Scars will be on the breast only and generally will be a straight horizontal line about four inches long.

This surgery is best suited for someone who does not want multiple scars or surgery that recruits skin, fat and tissue from a donor site. It's a great choice for someone who cannot decide on other breast reconstructions as this surgery preserves all donor sites and future options. It's also a great option for someone who had implants prior to being diagnosed with breast cancer and who prefers the look and feel of implants and also for someone who needs a quick recovery time.

This would not be a good choice for someone who does not want a foreign object implanted or someone who does not like the look of implants or someone who does not want to have replacement surgery every ten to fifteen years. I'd like to mention here that there are specific risks and complications inherent to this type of reconstructive surgery; capsular contracture, rupture, wrinkling, asymmetry, pain, possible infection, rejection and exposure of the implant.

If this surgery is done on its own, it's outpatient. If done immediately following a mastectomy, there is usually a twenty-three hour stay post-op. Recovery time needed is one to two weeks and there is a lifting restriction of no more than five pounds with the arm on the reconstructed side.

There will be drains in the breast only and they will be removed when, you guessed it, fluid total is 30cc's or less for a twenty-four hour period for two consecutive days. Depending on your plastic surgeon's preference you may be discharged wearing a "lovely" surgical bra or you may be asked to wear loose tops or a camisole for about three weeks.

Again, depending on your plastic surgeon's preference, expansions will begin the second or third week post-op.

One Step Gel Implant Reconstruction

This surgery involves skipping the tissue expander placement and going directly to reconstruction using the gel implant.

The ideal candidate for this surgery is someone who wants bilateral prophylactic mastectomies because of a strong family history of breast cancer or because they are BRCA positive gene carriers who do not have any active breast cancer. And someone who's nipples are in a good position and not ptotic or drooping.

This is a great option for someone, who in addition to the above, wants to be the same size as they are presently or slightly smaller and who does not mind some asymmetry as second stage revisions are usually not done .

All other general information is the same as for the tissue expander to gel implant reconstruction surgery.

Speaking of Revisions

Would you like some more really good news? First the breast cancer will be addressed and then you will have either immediate or delayed reconstruction. This is where the breast mound will be created. Now, here comes the great part.

The second stage of breast reconstruction will address both the revision of the reconstructed breast and the symmetry procedure for the non-cancer breast or if you have opted for bilateral mastectomies and reconstruction, then this second stage will address bilateral revisions.

Are you ready? Quite often this second stage will involve either fat grafting or liposuction or both ... "silver lining", of course, this will be determined by your plastic surgeon. Liposuction will remove fat from your donor sites, which is your abdomen, your back, your butt, and your thigh to create balance and proportion and fat grafting involves using liposuction to remove fat from where you don't want it to the places on your reconstructed breast where you need more fullness for symmetry.

Isn't that really good news? This is why breast reconstructive surgeons have some of the happiest patients. When all is said and done, most ladies look better after their reconstruction than before they were diagnosed with breast cancer. Seeing our ladies go through the whole process from breast cancer

Bernadette Hanson

diagnosis to being very happy with their "new normal" is one of the best things about my job as a nurse working in reconstructive surgery.

NOTES

Section 4

Some Parting Thoughts

I mentioned earlier that one of my favorite doctors says that the breasts are sisters and not twins, this bears repeating as you will tend to focus on them before, during and after reconstruction. This is quite a normal response for anyone that has gone through breast cancer. My point here is that your breasts were not perfectly symmetrical and positioned before reconstruction and they won't be after the reconstruction.

Of course, if you notice a new lump or bump, this should be addressed by your breast surgeon immediately. Or, if you notice any new irregularities on your reconstructed breasts, particularly breasts reconstructed with implants, this should be immediately addressed by your plastic surgeon.

Remember that scarring at the operative sites is normal and inevitable. A good portion of the scarring on the reconstructed breast will be concealed by the tattooing and reconstructed nipple. Also, it's important to be patient between the stages of breast reconstruction. There's a reason why it takes time to heal and resolve swelling and why the stages go in a specific order. If you were building an ice cream sundae you wouldn't put the cherry on the bottom, right? Each stage goes in order to give you the best possible result, so please be patient and trust your plastic surgeon.

Bernadette Hanson

Always follow your doctor's post-op instructions carefully to avoid complications and to achieve optimal results. This will usually include information outlining the signs and symptoms of infection, as well as detailed instructions regarding activities, diet, wound care, restrictions, and contact information for the person(s) to call in an emergency during office hours and nights and weekends.

I promised you a list of the most important questions to ask your plastic surgeon and some websites for breast cancer support groups.

Questions to Ask Your Plastic Surgeon

- Are you certified by the American Board of Plastic Surgery?
- What areas were you trained specifically in the field of plastic reconstructive surgery?
- Which breast reconstructive options am I a good candidate for?
- Which breast reconstructive option would you recommend for me?
- How many of these procedures have you done?
- What are the benefits, risks, and complications of that procedure?
- Where and how will you perform my procedure?
- How long of a recovery period can I expect and what kind of help will I need?
- What will be expected of me to get the best results?
- How are complications handled?
- Who do I call in case something happens after office hours or on the weekend?
- What are my options if I am dissatisfied with my results?
- Do you have before and after photos that I can look at?
- Can I talk with some of your patients who have had this same procedure done?

During your consultation with your plastic surgeon you can expect the following; an evaluation of your general health including pre-existing health conditions and risk factors; an examination of your breasts with measurements being taken as well as documenting breast size, shape, skin quality; placement of areola and nipples; and baseline pre-operative photos will be taken. There will be a discussion of options and a recommendation of a course of treatment as well as a conversation regarding likely outcomes of breast reconstruction; and any risks and potential complications.

Websites You need to Check Out

Here are some of the best and well established websites for anyone wanting to know more about breast cancer or for anyone with breast cancer seeking support and encouragement;

www.y-me.org

www.gildasclub.org

www.cancersupportcenter.org

www.cancerwellness.org

www.wellnesshouse.org

www.breastreconstruction.org

www.cancer.org

These websites contain information and contacts for one on one support, group support, free programs and resources, trained counselors, classes, networking, workshops, education, social activities, peer support from other breast cancer survivors, resources for wigs and breast prosthesis, and much more.

My hope is that you have found the information in this book to be informative, uplifting and helpful. I wish you well on your breast reconstruction journey and would like you to know that a portion of each sale of this book is going to Y-me.org for breast cancer resources, support and information.

I would love for you to visit the website:

www.myreconoptions.com and share your comments, insights, questions and victories.

Many blessings and stay encouraged,

b

Bernadette Hanson's Bio

She has been a registered nurse for almost 20 years and has been working in plastic surgery since 1997. She has worked exclusively in breast cancer reconstruction since 2005.

Her calling and her passion is to reach out to women with breast cancer through nursing care, education and implementation of each individual's treatment plan.

INDEX OF MEDICAL TERMS

- **Acellular dermis:** processed and purified donated skin used to support the tissue expander and gel implant
- **Areola:** pigmented skin surrounding the nipple
- **Atrophy:** to shrink, become smaller over time
- **Augmentation:** making a breast bigger, using an implant
- **Autologous tissue:** using tissue from various sites on your own body for breast reconstruction
- **Breast Biopsy:** outpatient test that involves removing a small sample of a suspected cancer , usually by needle and syringe
- **Breast prosthesis:** flexible breast form custom made that fits into a pocket on a mastectomy bra, used for symmetry while wearing clothing
- **Breast Surgeon:** the doctors that perform breast biopsies, lumpectomies, mastectomies
- **Capsular contracture:** hardening of the area inside the breast around implant or tissue expander
- **Completion Mastectomy:** removing the remainder of breast tissue after a lumpectomy has already been done
- **Delayed reconstruction:** breast reconstruction done as a separate surgery after the mastectomy and or treatments (chemo or radiation)
- **Donor site:** the area on your body where tissue has been taken to create your new breast (abdomen, thigh, buttock, back area)
- **Genetic Counselors :** the doctors that plan tests for you based on hereditary factors/inherited family conditions

- **Hematoma:** blood pooling beneath the skin
- **Holistic:** Caring for someone not only as far as the physical body, but also the intellect/mind and the emotions
- **Immediate reconstruction:** breast reconstruction done at the same time as the mastectomy
- **Implant reconstruction:** a two staged breast reconstruction process using tissue expanders first, then exchanging for gel implants
- **Lumpectomy:** surgical excision of a breast lump with some surrounding tissue
- **Mastopexy:** surgically lifting a breast to make it more youthful looking
- **Necrotizing fasciitis:** severe soft tissue infection, also called "skin eating" disease
- **Nipple Sparing Mastectomy:** removing the inner breast tissue and leaving the nipple and areola
- **Oncologist:** the doctors that plan chemo treatment
- **Oncoplastic reconstruction:** breast tissue rearrangement after a lumpectomy or partial mastectomy and before radiation treatment.
- **Partial Mastectomy:** larger than a lumpectomy and smaller than a mastectomy, this involves removing approximately 25% of the breast
- **Pathologist:** the doctors that look at tissue and fluid samples
- **Plastic Surgeons:** The doctors who will reconstruct your breast(s)
- **Plastic Surgery:** surgery to repair/replace/reform/restore/reshape injured, missing, or deformed parts of the body due to birth defects, disease process, burns and trauma

- **Prophylactic mastectomy:** preventative, risk reducing mastectomy on a breast that does not have cancer
- **Psych-Oncologist:** A therapist specially trained to help you through the emotional/psychological issues of breast cancer
- **Ptosis:** drooping of the breast due to the natural aging process
- **Radiation Oncologist:** the doctors that plan radiation treatment
- **Radical Mastectomy:** removing all inner breast tissue , including nipple and areola as well as lymph nodes and other surrounding tissues
- **Radiologist:** the doctors that take and interpret X-rays/images
- **Reduction:** surgically removing tissue and skin to make a breast smaller
- **Revision surgery:** second stage surgery that tweaks/adjusts/modifies/improves previous reconstructive work
- **Sentinel Node Biopsy:** surgical excision of lymph nodes under the arm / axilla
- **Seroma:** fluid pooling beneath the skin
- **Simple Mastectomy:** removing the inner breast tissue, areola and nipple
- **Social Workers:** professionals that evaluate your support system at home and plan for needed care/equipment when you are discharged from the hospital
- **Staging:** pre-surgery testing that determines exactly what type of breast cancer is present and how far it has spread.

- **Symmetry procedure:** surgery that addresses the non-cancer breast to make it similar in shape/size/projection to the reconstructed breast
- **Tattooing/medical micropigmentation:** sub dermal placement of ink to replace the color for the areola and nipple

www.ingramcontent.com/pod-product-compliance
Lightning Source LLC
Chambersburg PA
CBHW072152020426
42334CB00018B/1965